The Power of Health

Making Your Body Feel Rich

Author: Jay and Kavita

Introduction

Health is Life.

Being healthy is more than not being sick or having less illness. It is about being fit, having the energy and the strength to achieve life goals.

When we are down with sickness and disease, we start to regret not being able to live a healthy life. It is in our nature to regret something when things go down.

We almost eat as if we don't care about the future. And that's the problem. We can't deny the fact that we have this unreasonable craving for junk food as it tastes really good. However, junk food, dairy products, and processed meat are literally destroying our bodies slowly. I still get shocked sometimes when I hear people that I know that their relatives get cancer, or they themselves do. Why did it happen to them? And I thought that it might happen to me too if I didn't take a serious turn with my health.

Yes, we are in charge of our own health and that explains why people cause their own diseases because of the way they eat and live. Eating a lot of meat and dairy is far more dangerous than smoking. The unhealthier food we put in our body; the more things could go wrong.

We ignore the risk of eating and living healthily as we are hung up on "living only once and living the life to the fullest". Life is precious, why risk it?

Start living a healthy life, prepare to start now!

Why Health is Important?

Whatever you have achieved now or whatever you want to achieve in your life, it is your mind and body that is responsible to let it happen. If you want to lead your life instead of just living it, you must prioritize your health.

Health has three components:

Physical - Exercise is so pivotal when it comes to your personal life. A numerous studies and researches have shown that individuals who exercise on a regular basis have a better quality of life and can live longer as compared to those who don't.

Nutrition - Having proper nutrition is truly significant as far as health is concerned. Our body requires nutrition such as vitamins, protein, fat, minerals, etc. in order for it to function efficiently. It will also help to strengthen the immunity of our body. With a good immune system, it protects our body from diseases and eventually helps in avoiding future medical expenses.

Physiological - Without getting enough relaxation and rest, our body is going to start functioning inefficiently. Along with that, our performance will decrease too. There are a lot of complications that may arise at such times. This is where getting enough and proper sleep helps. Relaxing between physical activities helps.

The feeling of having complete physical, mental and social well-being is the best reward in maintaining good health. Living with the practice of a healthy lifestyle can prevent us from long-term illnesses like asthma, heart diseases, diabetes, and many more. It will definitely provide us the freedom from almost all diseases. It is very vital to maintain a healthy lifestyle for us to be fit and fearless of diseases. Eating healthy food and doing regular physical exercises are the key factors to stay fit. When you are healthy, you are happy. And happy life means a stress-free and disease-free life.

If an individual stays healthy physically, then that individual will stay healthy mentally too. Mental and physical health are linked primarily. If we stay fit and healthy by eating the right food and exercising regularly, our body will help us to deal with daily stress.

The body cells are made up of different chemical substances and they move from one place to another. Moreover, several other activities are happening in our body that our body needs, which are, energy and raw material. For our body cells and tissues to function well, food is essential. To live fit and healthy, good nutrition is a must and we should make a habit of it.

It is said, "Health is wealth". If health is lost, everything is lost. If you are not healthy, then your capacity to work will be poor. Incapability to work will lead to poverty and misery. For a normal individual, health is the absence of sickness and diseases. That view is frail and one-sided. The word or term "health" is much more comprehensive. Good health is the state of all-around well-being of a person. It will enable a person to live and work normally and to resist the negative impact of the environment.

It is, therefore, crucial to maintaining good health. You cannot buy good health; you should work for it. Acquiring good health requires certain steps. According to doctors and specialists, three basic factors bring about good health - a clean environment, good habits, and a clean mind.

The Benefits of Good Health

 Eat healthily and properly. Sleep well. Exercise regularly. This seems to be the cycle of the current generation. Undeniably, a lot of this generation is born with body image issues, and the need to look their best at all times is their priority. However, maintaining good health is not just about physical appearance, it is about being healthy overall. If you are living your life with good food, proper exercise, sleep, and enough fluids, then the result will be a positive effect on your physical appearance, mental and even emotional health. In this chapter, let's discuss the benefits of having good health:

You will be active and energetic.

That is definitely true. Living a moderately healthy life, you will be more active and energetic; living your life with a lot of vigor. Most of us have been through phrases made by long hours of work, unhealthy eating schedules and a little to fewer hours of sleep. Having gone through that phase, we become lethargic or drowsy throughout the day. It will take serious negative effects on our emotional and rational capabilities. It is crucial for us to get about 8 hours of sleep with a balanced diet and at least 30 minutes of exercise of any kind.

Good medical records.

Studies have shown that individuals who eat healthy food and doing regular exercise are at lower risk of contracting illnesses such as arthritis, diabetes, asthma, cardiovascular problems, etc. Physical exercise helps in regulating blood flow in our body. It also balances our metabolism that boosts our overall health. A proper diet and regular exercise transcend to low cholesterol, a leaner body, and strong immunity.

You will be more confident.

When we are not feeling our best, our confidence will go down with it too. But if we are living a healthy life for a while now, we feel that confidence within. We know that we look good. You will have that healthy glow that good food and exercise give us. We are clear-minded, which means that we are ready to take future challenges. We are also aware that we will perform well in whatever we are assigned. Having a positive self-awareness will make us more confident and we will continuously do better on a daily basis.

Emotional stability.

It is not a surprising fact that mood is a lot psychosomatic or psychological. Have you ever felt good whenever you went out in the cold and you didn't stop sneezing and retching? No, right? Well, that is because when our body doesn't feel good, our mind does not either. Mood swings are unavoidable with hormonal ups and downs. However, we can definitely limit them to certain periods. A balanced diet, lots of fluids, regular exercise, and enough sleep boost the release of serotonin or the happy hormone. Although a sweet treat and alcohol will give us a temporary spike in our happy hormones, a healthy habit will guarantee that high for the longer-term.

Better looking.

Salty chips, fatty foods, carbonated drinks, and an immoderate amount of sugar will make us feel great on the taste buds and will give us a glow of happiness. But wait, that is not all. Those kinds of foods will give us wrinkles, extra padding on the belly, and the lethargic pace that comes with carrying around excess weight. A proper and healthy diet which consists of fruits, vegetables, grains, lots of water intake, enough sleep and a good amount of exercise will get rid of that unwanted belly fat. It will also keep your skin glowing and your hair shiny. A healthy habit will reflect on our body and movements; leaving us more supple and attractive.

Productivity.

As I mentioned at the beginning of this chapter, a healthier lifestyle will keep you more active and energetic. With enough sleep, you will not feel fatigued throughout the day. Cutting down your alcohol intake also means that you won't risk a hangover. Smoking and caffeine will give you a temporary spike in energy, but eventually, they will make you tired in the long run. A healthy lifestyle will keep our minds clear and our bodies fit. You won't feel sleepy. You won't feel sick. You will be ready to take the day in an energetic and productive manner.

They say that old habits die hard. Quitting bad habits may be impossible, but it will never be too late to start a healthy lifestyle. Take in lots of greens and fiber in your diet with lots of water and fruits. Cut down on unhealthy snacks and cigarettes. As far as our health is concerned, little steps will go a long way.

How Does Food Impact Our Health?

We are all aware that eating healthy is beneficial and can help prevent disease. Numerous studies show that eating rich and healthy food provides us good nutrients that will let our body reach its full potential. Along with that, it also supports the immune system that protects us from illness and disease. But how does our diet actually impact our health?

The food we input into our body gives "information" and materials it needs to function properly. And if we don't get the right information, our metabolic processes will suffer and our health will decline. If we consume too much food that gives our body the wrong information, then we become overweight, undernourished and we will be at great risk of developing illness and diseases.

In short, what we eat is what controls our health. Food acts as the medicine that maintains, prevents, and treats disease.

What does food do in our bodies?

The nutrient in our food intake enables the cell in our body to do their necessary functions. This just simply describes that the nutrients present in the food are essential for our body to function.

The nutrients in our body are the nourishing substances that are essential for the development, growth, and maintenance of our body functions. It means that if a nutrient is not present, the aspect of function is will not, therefore, human health will decline. If the nutrient we intake does not meet the nutrient our body needs, our metabolic processes will slow down or even stop.

In other words, the nutrients will give our body the fuel to function. With this, food serves as the source of "information" for the body. Thinking about food in this sense will give us the view of the nutrition that goes beyond calories or grams, good food or bad food. This will lead us to focus on what food we should include in our diet rather than the food we should exclude.

As an alternative, instead of viewing food as the enemy, we need to focus on viewing food as a way to help our body maintain its function.

Food Issues

Processing removes nutrients

Supermarkets offer a variety of convenient packaged foods that are appealing to our taste buds. However, these packaged foods compromise our nutrition. Most of these foods' natural nutrients are removed in the process. Hence, we need to get them elsewhere.

Processed foods have additives

Most of us rely heavily on processed foods that include additives, flavorings, artificial colorings, and chemically-altered fats and sweeteners. These additives may be giving our bodies the wrong signals or information instead of the information our bodies need to function properly.

Some "natural" foods have fewer nutrients

Foods from past years are not the same currently. The nutrients in the soil have been depleted, therefore, the food in that solid only contains fewer nutrients. Nowadays, chemicals are mostly used in raising both animals and plants, specifically on large industrial farms.

Less variety of foods

Unfortunately, while many new food products are being introduced each year, two-thirds of our calories come from just four foods which are rice, corn, soy, and wheat.

Eating for convenience

In our fast-paced and modern society, we tend to eat for convenience instead of health and pleasure. Fast foods remove the pleasure of creating and savoring an amazing meal. It also prevents us from connecting and enjoying a good slow meal.

What is the connection between food and disease?

Society is facing significant health problems. This has a major effect on productivity because of chronic health issues.

Various researches believed that these issues are partly related to diet. While they used to believe that chronic diseases were caused by a single gene mutation, they are now considering that these attributes to a network of biological dysfunction. Not surprisingly, the food we eat is a crucial factor in that dysfunction because our diets lack the necessary nutrients needed.

To prevent the start of these diseases, we need to know how various nutrients in our diet interrelate and affect our body's functions.

How Your Eating Habits Affect Our Health

It's a given fact that when we eat healthy food, we become healthy. But how does the food we take have such a huge effect on how we function on a daily basis?

We are aware that when it comes to our health, the food we intake has a significant effect, particularly when it comes to our heart. Stress, weight gain, physical inactivity, obesity, high blood pressure, and high cholesterol can significantly increase the risks of heart diseases and various cancers.

The food we input into our body serves as the information and fuel it needs for our body to properly function. If our body does not get the right information, the metabolic processes can suffer and our health can decline. It is important to have good nutrition based on healthy eating habits to enable you to stay healthy, active, and live a longer life.

In short, the nutrition we put in our body helps us to avoid certain diseases that can put our life at risk and cause our health to deteriorate.

Our eating habit is a combination of our physiological and psychological aspect. Physically, an individual tends to overeat due to malfunctioning of the hunger and appetite hormones. This usually happens due to major nutrient deficiencies or undernourishment. It is where our body craves for sugar. Another part of this can be dehydration, which is often misinterpreted as hunger.

Psychologically, our eating habits are affected by the sleep-wake cycle, mood swings, anxiety, peer pressure, excitement or depression.

Nutrition and Disease

When we eat, the food we intake goes through a digestive process. This part of this process involves absorbing minerals and vitamins from that food and distributing it into the bloodstream which centers on the heart muscle, coronary arteries, and blood vessels.

Our heart can pump harder and exert more energy depending on what type of food we are going to input into our body. This could lead to heart failure and heart attack. Our sodium intake has a major role in affecting our heart rate and blood pressure. When we consume salty foods, our body will retain water to dilute the blood volume. This will cause more blood to circulate throughout our body and our heart to work harder.

The recommended sodium intake as instructed by the Centers for Disease Control and Prevention is 180 – 150 mg of sodium in a day. However, on average, we consume over 3,400 mg of sodium in a day. Blame it to those pre-prepared and processed foods.

A diet that is high in saturated and trans fats will raise our bad cholesterol that could lead to the hardenings of arteries and plaque forming on the inner linings of our blood vessels which will further narrow them. Those narrowed openings can mean that as the heart receives the blood, it must work harder to maintain blood flow in order to pump blood through the narrowed openings.

Correspondingly, if we are not maintaining a healthy diet this could increase our risk for various cancers. A study published in 2018, states that the amount of processing and the amount of change the ingredients go through to help improve the coloring, flavor, and shelf life. It was found that every 10% increase in consumption of processed foods was linked with a 12% higher risk for cancer overall and an 11% increased risk for breast cancer.

Whereas these foods can cause harm, there are foods that can help to improve our health and heart function. Healthy fats like olive oil and whole grains help in lowering our cholesterol and help prevent plaque from forming in the arteries. As the blood flow improves, our heart will be able to pump blood easier that will cause less strain and stress on our heart which could ultimately lower our heart rate.

Poor Nutrition

When our body is deprived of the nourishment it needs, that can lead to poor nutrition and bad eating habits which basically causes obesity, diabetes, and can increase the risk of other chronic diseases such as heart disease, stroke, and cancer.

The source of poor nutrition is our intake of unhealthy and wrong types of food. These types of food do not have the nutrients that our body needs the most. They are fundamentally low in fiber and vitamins or high in fat, salt, and sugar. Although a lot of packaged foods we purchase at the supermarkets meet our taste bud requirements, these packaged and stored food may strip off the nutrients our body requires and eliminate our chance of a healthier lifestyle.

Poor nutrition is also caused by overeating. Taking in more calories than what we are burning each day, even if these foods are the foods, it can eventually result in weight gain and can lead to obesity. Overweight and obesity can lead to diabetes and heart diseases.

On the other side, undereating deprives our body of the nutrients it needs. Individuals who suffer from diseases such as bulimia and anorexia are just as much at the risk of heart complications and diseases as those who overeat.

If you are anxious about the number of calories you are putting in your body on a daily basis, it is best to discuss with your doctor or health experts.

How does poor nutrition affect our health?

Poor nutrition can affect our health in many ways, not only can it lead to chronic illnesses and diseases, but it can also affect our mental health, complexion, energy levels, and our overall well-being. Poor nutrition contributes to stress, exhaustion, and our productivity towards work. Additionally, it can lead to:

- being overweight or obese
- tooth decay
- high blood pressure

- high cholesterol
- heart disease and stroke
- type-2 diabetes
- osteoporosis
- some cancers
- depression
- eating disorders

Poor nutrition can damage our overall wellbeing and reduce our ability to lead a happy and active life.

Unhealthy Eating Habits

We, humans, are creatures of habit. We like buying the same foods from the same store. We prepare the same recipes time and again. We live within our own daily routines. The problem is that we get so comfortable in our routines and we are having a hard time giving up old habits.

A lot of us are hesitant about changing our diets because we have grown accustomed to eating or drinking the same foods regularly. Even when we want to change, old habits really die hard. In the course of time, our habits become automatic, learned behaviors, and these factors are stronger to incorporate than trying new habits into our lives.

At times, even if we manage to change our bad eating habits, we easily fall back on our old ways in times of stress. When we are in a vulnerable state, our automatic responses often override good intentions.

The bad stuff, sugars, fats, salts, etc. will kill you sooner or later. Gaining fat around the heart (as the central body) will do terrible things to our health.

All of these bad things are essential to our existence, but too much of them are detrimental to our health. Our ancestors needed these things to provide the energy to allow us t exist. But now, we are almost powerless to resist these bad habits.

Unhealthy eating habits are not established purposely sometimes, however, these habits affect our health. The side effects of these habits include:

Skipping Breakfast

Some of us, if not most of us would be surprised that skipping breakfast is included in unhealthy eating habits. When we skip our breakfast, our body is starving for 12- 18 hours, and when we will consume our first meal that it would be rich and our body will store that food in the form of fat that can result in obesity.

Binge Eating

Binge eating is done when you are out for a party or while having that movie marathon you have been looking forward to. Mostly binging is done with junk food which is rich in fat, salt, sugar, and calories. These junk foods are addicting as they taste good, but these are the major player to cause obesity, high blood sugar levels, elevated cholesterol levels, high blood pressure, fatty liver, and other diseases.

Snacking on unhealthy foods

We often feel hungry after that long day we spend at work and the want to grab anything on the way to fill our stomach is eminent. This is a crucial time to be mindful of what should we put in our body rather than mindlessly eating anything we set our eyes to. Unhealthy eating, which is mostly composed of junk foods, leads to obesity, high blood sugar levels, elevated cholesterol levels, high blood pressure, and fatty liver.

Eating too quickly

When we swallow our food, whether we are snacking or eating or regular meal, it doesn't give our brain time to comprehend that we are already full. Our brain will not send the signal that we are full until about 15 - 20 minutes after we have started eating. That said, we have to chew our food properly. If we eat too quickly or too fast, this might lead to acidity, bloating weight gain and etc.

However, if you want to live a healthier life, you need to shake it up a bit and change those bad eating habits. Start thinking in a different way about your diet and lifestyle. For us to stay fit, we have to be mindful of our eating habits to avoid adverse effects on our health.

Why Should We Avoid Unhealthy Eating Habits?

Anything that promises short-cuts is most probably a sham. Some may work at first, but they are rarely sustainable and successful for the long term. Some may cause more harm than good.

Here are some of the reasons why we should avoid unhealthy eating habits:

Nutrition Deficiency

Some fad diets focus on eliminating something. There numerous fad diets that promise quick results. Some of these fad diets focus on eliminating something. If you have tried a diet that asked you to cut off your carbs, fat, liquid diets, eat only specific foods, or anything extreme, that diet is not really healthy for you. Our body needs balance so that we can get all the minerals, vitamins, and nutrients we need to function properly.

These diets that revolve around consuming an only specific type of food, like only fat, only raw eggs, slimming pills, slimming tea, or only cabbages, are unhealthy for the same reason as above. It causes nutrition deficiency.

Fatigued or stressed

Missing out on certain meals will make us extremely hungry or thirsty. This will not only deprive us of the nutrients that our body needs, but it will also cause us fatigue and stress. When we are stressed out, our body produces a certain hormone which is cortisol. When the level of cortisol increases, it causes the insulin level to rise. Our blood sugar then will drop causing us to crave sugary and unhealthy food.

Slowing down of Metabolism

Starving yourself will only result in to slow metabolism. If we consume a little number of calories or deprive ourselves of a balanced diet, our body will work to preserve the little resources we take by going into starvation mode. So, instead of burning fat, our body will hold on to it for the energy and fuel it needs.

Instead of thinking of ways to cut down our food intake to avoid overeating and gaining weight, we should focus on what we should eat. The best way is to change our unhealthy eating habits. Choose a lifestyle that you can enjoy and you can keep for the long term.

Healthy Eating Habits

We are all aware that healthy eating can transform our lives and help us live a long and happy one. But what does healthy eating entails? How do we start putting this into practice and break the bad habits? Some of us may take this as a way to lose extra weight, others may take this as a way to keep their blood pressure low, the remaining others may take this as their way of living healthier.

However, this transformation doesn't happen overnight. You can't just wake up the next morning and break all your bad habits. This is a slow and steady process. Here are some helpful tips that will help you have a healthy eating habit:

Eat more fruits and vegetables. Change your unhealthy snacks to a serving of fruits. Have a bowl of oatmeal or cereals with some berries on it. Aim for a serving of fruits and veggies in a day.

Eat less saturated and trans fats. Check the labels of the products that you are buying. Be mindful of the ingredients and opt for the better and healthy ones.

Eat less salt. Avoid stocking up on your favorite chips. Make an effort in putting less salt on your food.

Eat less sugar. You may substitute sugar with honey in your morning coffee. You may also opt for less sugary treats and desserts.

Increase intake of fiber. Stock up on fiber-rich foods such as millet, vegetables, nuts, fruits, whole grains, and oats. These foods are known to curb hunger in the most healthy and nutritious way. It will make you satiated and will trim down weight as well.

Drink more water. Avoid sugary and colored drinks and choose water instead. Drinking a lot of water can help you lose weight and can clear your complexion. Dehydration is often misunderstood as being hungry. So, drinking enough water can control our bad eating habits.

Check your portions. Check the portion of food on your plate before digging in. It is better if you have a portion of vegetables and a portion of lean protein like meat, chicken, fish, or legumes in a quarter space of your plate. On the other half quarter of your plate, add in your grains like rice, noodles or pasta. Make sure to use a smaller plate. The size of your plate affects the portioning of your food. Consumption from a smaller plate can influence the brain to release the appetite hormone which triggers a feeling of early fullness.

Plan ahead. Meal planning and having a list of food to buy are the best ways to avoid stocking up on unhealthy and preserved packaged goods. One of the reasons why we end up eating fast food is because we are in a rush. Plan out your meals over the weekends then buy the necessary ingredients to prepare your food. This will not only help you eat healthily; it will also help you save money.

Maintain a good sleeping routine. An interrupted sleep cycle can cause us to crave and eat salty foods due to loss of energy. It also hinders the functioning of individual organs, due to which the body demands more calories to work. This is a common symptom of obesity.

Staying Healthy

What is the best way to stay healthy?

A healthy body and will increase your productivity especially at work. There are several ways available for us to keep our body fit and healthy. Here are my simple yet powerful tips that you can follow if you want for a healthier life:

BODY

Eat Right.

If your gut is well and healthy, only then you can eat and get the nutrition required for any kind of physical changes in your body. Our gut affects our mood, so, we should keep it balanced.

Invest in whole foods such as fruits, vegetables, grains (brown rice, whole grain oats), bread, and raw nuts and seeds. Eating these whole foods will help you control the portion of food intake because all the fiber will make you feel full and will prevent you from overeating. Their nutrient density prevents cravings.

Stock up on high-quality meats and seafood that you can reasonably afford. Add healthy fats like coconut, avocado, fish and meat, and butter to the list. Avoid refined carbohydrates, sugar, and trans fats. These kinds of food ingredients basically lead to diabetes, obesity, cancer, and heart disease.

Eat sweets in moderation. If you are craving something sweet, avoid refined added sugar and opt for some frozen or fresh fruit but not fruit juice.

Cook your meals from scratch and choose fresh and raw ingredients. Avoid unnecessary ingredients and additives such as sugar, preservatives, flavor enhancers, unhealthy fats, and food colors. If you want to eat processed foods, choose only the ones with no added sugar and with limited ingredients. Always read labels carefully.

Eat Light.

Our body requires much less than we eat, so, we should be aware of what we put in our body. Avoid spicy and takeout food. Try to have your dinner as early as possible and have a gap of at least 2–3 hours in your dinner and sleep time. It is better to have small meals in-between main meals so that you will not overeat. You can eat fruit, veggies, or nuts for snacks. Avoid colored and flavored drinks.

Drink lots of water.

Drink plenty of water and hydrate yourself. It is better to drink a glass of warm water as soon as you get up in the morning. Do not eat anything for at least 40-60 minutes after drinking. It will be better if you will add a little honey to it as it gives positive energy and helps in little lubrication. If you do this for a couple of weeks, you will see a huge difference in the quality of your mornings.

Just before every meal, drink a glass of water. When you drink a glass of water before eating, you will feel a little full and will not be tempted to overeat.

Drinking a lot of water has its benefits:

- It lubricates the joints.
- It forms saliva which helps in digesting food and keeps the mouth, nose, and eyes moist. It also keeps our mouths clean.
- It increases skin health and beauty.
- It regulates body temperature.
- It keeps balancing in the digestive system.
- Water is needed to flush out body waste like urine and feces.
- It helps to maintain blood pressure.

Kidney regulates fluid in the body so that a sufficient amount of water can't lead to kidney stones and other problems and prevents the kidney damage.

Minimize caffeine.

Replace coffee and tea with herbal teas, because caffeine also triggers the release of stress hormones. If you will notice, you feel alert after a strong cup of tea or coffee, why? Because the stress hormones suppress sleep. If you are used to your daily fix of caffeine to get you through the day, you need to understand that you are tired and sleepy. A human body needs rest to repair and rejuvenate the body tissues. A well-rested body performs better. A human body would not need a rush of adrenaline for energy to get through the day if you could only give what it truly needs and craves, proper nutrition and rest. When you really think about it, caffeine is actually no help at all if you get that.

Sleep.

I bet you've heard this one before. Try to get at least 8 hours most nights. I know that you won't regularly have this privilege of 8 hours of sleep, but if you make it a priority, you can do this most of the time. Sleep right as our body needs rest to heal itself and be healthy. Focus on getting proper sleep every day. Avoid all of your electronic devices for at least 15 minutes before going to sleep. Focus on getting sleep, think positive.

Sleeping helps the body and mind to restore and regenerate and it's very essential to our overall physical and mental health. When we lack sleep, our stress hormones rise which will have a negative effect on our mood.

Getting sufficient sleep is one of the most significant life hacks that is largely ignored today. When we sleep well, we become stronger, more focused, motivated, happy, and clear-minded. All these qualities contribute to our achievements in other areas of our lives. Sleeping also improves the brain's functionality hence creativity.

Exercise.

Exercise or physical activities help improve blood circulation, increase metabolism, brain function, and other body systems in general. Ideally, 3 - 4 times a week of doing certain exercises really help.

Don't be overly inactive. Get up and move. Take a walk. Use the stairs instead of the elevator. Use the other bathroom, the one that is a little farther away. This is not supposed to be to be a form of exercise. This is just to get you up and moving around. Set a timer if it helps.

You can do weights once per week and occasional sprints. Some people think they need to exercise multiple times a day to burn more calories. That is up to you but make sure that you won't strain your muscles. Do what works for you.

Health is more important than fitness. Work out for health at least if not fitness. The difference between If the focus is long-term health, go for medium-level activities, like walks, jogs, yoga, lightweights, and core activities. Free body exercises are the best such as doing morning yoga which can actually affect almost all parts of your life and removing many diseases. There are a lot of free videos on YouTube which you can choose from.

Stress Management.

Practice stress management. Stress is one of the main reasons for unhealthy weight and disease. Stress releases cortisol that converts fuel sources into glucose (sugar) because the body needs the energy to respond. Cortisol transforms stored fuel from different parts of the body such as muscles that leads to a decrease in lean body mass which causes the metabolic rate to fall. Since our current stress is usually non-life threatening and a completely different, chronic kind of stress (such as work or finance), we do not need the available glucose, especially when taken from our muscle mass. Add this to our inactive lifestyle, the glucose does not get used up and instead is deposited as unwanted belly fat. This also causes our blood cholesterol levels to rise. Numerous studies have found that chronic stress can take a major toll on our body that contributes to reduced immunity, high blood pressure, heart disease, obesity, anxiety, and depression.

Don't drink alcohol and smoke.

Avoid drinking alcohol as much as possible. Certainly, social drinking in moderation is ok. Smoking is dangerous as well as drinking, and doing both is even worse. Alcohol and cigarettes characterize serious health risks to the public. Smoking a cigarette causes lung cancer, stroke, COPD, heart disease, and many other multiple health problems. Smoking has been called the leading cause of death in the world. While drinking is much more socially acceptable than smoking, it too brings serious health risks.

Drinking severely causes mouth, throat, and breast cancer, stroke, brain damage, heart disease, and liver disease. Although low-risk drinkers considerably reduce their risk of developing such health problems as a result of their drinking, no level of alcohol consumption can be safe. With plenty of risks associated with the individual substances, the fact that combining alcohol and tobacco creates an even bigger risk shouldn't come as much of a surprise. However, since these conditions have many risk factors (things that increase your risk of developing them), it can be difficult to estimate what the effect of combining smoking and drinking will be.

Minimize exposure to toxins and chemicals.

This is far more important than most of us realize. While it is nearly impossible to eliminate all chemicals from our lives, we can definitely minimize the chemicals we are exposed to, especially those in household products. We can always choose biodegradable and non-toxic options for cleaners, detergents, and personal care products we use at home. We absorb all these chemicals through our skin and inhale them, the liver then has to detoxify these chemicals, adding to its burden.

Laugh more.

Laughter reduces stress hormones such as cortisol, adrenaline, and dopamine and increases the levels of endorphins (feel-good hormones) which relieves stress. This contributes to a better and positive outlook in life.

Get regular checkups.

A regular medical check-up is vital for the benefit of your well-being and overall health. Visit your doctor quarterly or twice in a year. This will help you detect any possible health problems to be diagnosed or treated properly. Additionally, it can also help to diagnose possible diseases at an early stage where the chances for treatment and cure are higher.

Take multivitamins or supplements.

Vitamin deficiencies are commonly linked to chronic diseases and supplements can help. A complete diet may not be giving you the nutrients you need, that's where multivitamins come in.

A daily multivitamin can help provide a good foundation for your health and can also protect you when you're experiencing stress, sleeping poorly, or not getting regular exercise.

Here are some multivitamins and supplements that you can take to help boost the nutrients that our body needs:

Magnesium

Magnesium plays a vital role in keeping your body and mind healthy. This essential nutrient is known for being important to our bone health and energy production. Taking a magnesium supplement can help.

However, magnesium may have more benefits which are:

- calm our nervous system and reduce
- ease sleep problems
- regulate muscle and nerve function
- balance blood sugar levels

Some of us are magnesium deficient because we aren't eating the right foods, not because we need supplements. Try to eat more pumpkin, spinach, artichoke, soybeans, beans, tofu, brown rice, or nuts before taking supplements for solutions.

Vitamin D

Vitamin D has numerous roles in your body, including the regulation of a particular neurotransmitters. It also helps our body to absorb calcium which is essential for bone health If we are not getting enough of Vitamin D, it can increase:

- your likelihood of getting sick
- your chances of bone and back pain
- bone and hair loss

Foods with vitamin D:

- fatty fish
- egg yolks
- fortified foods like milk, juice, and cereal

Calcium

Calcium is known for providing our body the mineral it needs for having strong bones and teeth. Women specifically start to lose bone density in their earlier years and getting enough calcium from the start is the best defense.

Foods rich in calcium:

- fortified cereals
- milk, cheese, and yogurt
- salty fish
- broccoli and kale
- nuts and nut butter

- beans and lentils

If your diet consists of these foods, you are likely getting enough calcium in your body.

Zinc

Zinc helps in healing wounds. It also supports our immune system and helps the body to use carbohydrates, protein, and fat for energy

Foods rich in zinc:

- oysters
- grass-fed beef
- pumpkin seeds
- spinach
- organ meats
- tahini
- sardines
- brown rice
- wheat germ
- tempeh

Iron

Iron is a multivitamin that helps increase energy, better brain function, and healthy red blood cells.

Food rich in iron:

- spinach
- shellfish
- liver
- legumes
- red meat
- pumpkin seeds

* quinoa
* broccoli
* tofu

Ginkgo Biloba

Ginkgo biloba is a plant native to China that has been used for hundreds of years as a remedy for various health conditions. It also reduces stress and anxiety by lowering levels of cortisol.

Oregano Oil

Oregano oil has countless antioxidant and antibacterial properties due to its active ingredient, carvacrol. Oregano oil also acts as an antidepressant by increasing dopamine in our body.

Some of the potential benefits of oregano:

* Natural antibiotic
* May help lower cholesterol
* Powerful antioxidant
* Could help treat yeast infections
* May improve gut health
* May have anti-inflammatory properties
* Could help relieve pain
* May have cancer-fighting properties
* May help you lose weight

Fish Oil

Fish oil supplements mainly contain two types of omega-3 fatty acids - docosahexaenoic acid (DHA) and eicosatetraenoic acid (EPA). Omega-3 fatty acids are vital nutrients that are significant in stopping and dealing with heart diseases.

Omega-3 fatty acids may help to:

- Lower blood pressure
- Reduce triglycerides
- Slow the development of plaque in the arteries
- Reduce the chance of abnormal heart rhythm
- Reduce the likelihood of heart attack and stroke
- Lessen the chance of sudden cardiac death in people with heart disease

Folate

Folate or folic acid is known for aiding in fetus development and preventing birth defects. However, folic acid or folate can help with growing out nails, fighting depression, or looking to combat inflammation.

Foods rich in folate:

- dark leafy greens
- avocado
- beans
- citrus

Ginseng

Ginseng has been used in traditional Chinese medicine since ancient times and the root can be eaten raw or steamed, but it's also available in other forms, such as tea, capsules, or pills. Supported by studies and experiments, ginseng may enhance brain skills, including mood, behavior, and memory.

Vitamin B-12

The B-vitamin complex helps in breaking down the micronutrients we consume like fats, proteins, carbs. It also works to keep our body's nerve and blood cells healthy.

Foods with Vitamin B-12:

- sardines

- tuna
- salmon
- egg
- milk and dairy products

Ginger

Ginger is known as one of the oldest medicinal herbs and one of the world's most popular culinary spices. It is a powerful antioxidant and with anti-inflammatory properties that are mainly responsible for its healing power. Ginger suppresses inflammation, a risk factor for numerous brain-related conditions including depression. It also increases levels of important brain chemicals, including dopamine and serotonin.

When it comes to vitamins and supplements, we should get them from food first. It's best to consult with your doctor or healthcare provider before adding any vitamins and supplements to your daily routine. This is especially true if you have a medical condition or if you are on any medications. Our bodies are intended to reap nutrients from the food that we eat and we get the nutrients that we need as long as we are eating a balanced diet. Vitamins and supplements are considered bonus boosters, not replacements for food. provider before adding any vitamins and supplements to your daily routine. This is especially true if you have a medical condition or if you are on any medications. Our bodies are intended to reap nutrients from the food that we eat and we get the nutrients that we need as long as we are eating a balanced diet. Vitamins and supplements are considered bonus boosters, not replacements for food.

<u>MIND</u>

A mind can help you in achieving everything you want be it your career or fitness goals, so keep training it slowly without over-stressing it.

Relax

Have some time in the day when you just relax, like your body, your mind also needs to rest. Take small breaks during work, close your eyes and just relax. Don't overthink or stress yourself. Have realistic goals and plan for them. Do not overwhelm yourself.

Meditate

This is something that you can do to increase your focus levels. Find some time alone and meditate. The emptiness of thoughts is difficult to achieve but with proper practice, you can achieve it.

Benefits of meditating:

Meditation is not something you only do for a difficult time. However, when things suddenly changed radically around you, having the focus and awareness of how you are dealing with the realities of your daily life can help lessen the overwhelming negative emotions.

The practice of meditation is not about blocking out our feelings in stressful times, but it can pinpoint how certain trials can make you feel and how you carry those feelings throughout. As you practice mindfulness, meditation then can help you prioritize your thoughts, block out the negativity and will find positive things when the days are darker.

The proven benefits of meditation will include:

- Improved sleep
- Reduced anxiety
- Minimized stress
- Greater focus; less distraction
- Newfound gratitude
- Healthier work-life balance
- Anger management
- Positive body image
- Stronger relationships

- Boosted immune system

In fact, the CDC (Centers for Disease Control and Prevention) even recommends including meditation as a fundamental strategy to maintain our mental health, cope with stress, and taking care of your body.

Practice Meditation

All of us can practice meditation to boost our mental, physical and emotional health. Additionally, it is simple and can be done anywhere without the use of special equipment. Here's how to add meditation to your daily routine to protect your mental health during this time of the pandemic:

- You can start with 2 minutes daily because you will find it much easier to stick to your practice if you start with a short period of just 2minutes at first. This practice can be beneficial particularly in forming a habit that will last longer. If you feel like continuing this practice, you can then adjust the time gradually.
- Choose to sit or lie comfortably. You can basically sit on a pillow on the floor or you can sit on a chair or on a couch if you are not comfortable sitting on the floor.
- Close your eyes after you have found your comfortable position. If you opted to lie down, you can use cooling eye masks.
- Pay attention to your breathing. You have to focus on your breathing as you inhale and exhale through your nostrils. Breathe deeply and slowly and if you find your mind wandering, slowly return your focus to your breathing.
- Engage in prayer because prayer is the best known and most widely practiced example of meditation.

Read

Yes, read. Spare some time for reading every day. It will not only increase your knowledge it will also help you in focusing, and giving yourself some quality time. You will surely learn a lot which will help you in many ways and keep your mind healthy. Sets a very positive example for your family and kids.

Listen to music

Good music will always soothe up things. Close your eyes and let your mind feel the music and its power. It can calm your mind and create positive and satisfactory feeling which is very good for your mind.

Spend time with family and friends.

Spend time with your family and genuinely love them. If you are away from them, call them as often as you get. Your family and love ones always bring the feeling of positivity which is good for your mental health. Share your problems or issues with them if possible and they will always give you the most genuine solutions selflessly. Spend time with your friends too. Being socially active can also affect our mood in a positive result.

Yeah. I know. This is short but it states what's important. Taking up and mindfully watching out for these activities will the chance of living healthy.

List of Healthy Foods

It's easy to identify which food are the healthiest. The food we intake goes through different metabolic pathways in our body and they can have different effects on our hunger, hormones, and our mood which can affect our health.

Below are the most healthy-friendly foods:

Whole Eggs

Even if a high intake of eggs raises the levels of "bad" cholesterol in some of us, they are still one of the best foods to eat if you want to lose weight. Eggs are high in protein and fat and they are very satiating.

Leafy Green Veggies

Leafy greens such as spinach, kale, collards, swiss chards to name a few have several properties that make them perfect for losing weight. These greens are low in calories and carbohydrates and loaded with fiber that helps you keep feeling full. Eating green veggies is a good way to increase the volume of your meals without the worry of increasing the calories.

Salmon

Salmon is a fatty fish that is incredibly healthy and satisfying. It will keep you full for many hours with a few calories. This fish is loaded with high-quality protein, essential nutrients, and healthy fats. Fish supplies a significant amount of iodine that is necessary for proper thyroid function. This is important to keep our metabolism running properly. Salmon is also high in omega-3 fatty acids which help to reduce inflammation that plays a major role in obesity and other diseases.

Cruciferous Vegetables

Cruciferous vegetables are vegetables of the mustard family which include broccoli, cabbage, cauliflower, and Brussels sprouts. These vegetables are high in fiber and contain a decent amount of protein. These types of vegetables can keep you full too.

Lean Beef and Chicken Breast

Meat is a weight loss-friendly food because it's high in protein. Protein is the most fulfilling nutrient that our body needs. Eating a high-protein meal can help you burn up to 80–100 more calories. If you opted on a low-carb diet plan, feel free to eat fatty meats. But if you are on a moderate- to a high-carb diet, choose lean meats.

Tuna

Tuna is low in fat but a lean source of high-quality protein. This fish helps increase protein intake while keeping total calories and fat low. It is an effective weight loss strategy, especially on a calorie-restricted diet.

Beans and Legumes

Beans and legumes such as lentils, black beans, kidney beans, and some others tend to be high in protein and fiber. These two essential nutrients will lead to satiation and a lower calorie intake.

Avocados

Avocados are high in carbs, loaded with healthy fats, and also contain many essential nutrients, including fiber and potassium. However, ensure that you keep your intake in moderation.

Apple Cider Vinegar

A lot of health enthusiast uses apple cider vinegar as condiment or dressing on salads and meals. Some people even dilute it in water to drink. Vinegar helps reduce blood sugar spikes after meals which may have various health benefits in the long run

Nuts

Nuts containing balanced amounts of protein, fiber, and healthy fats. However, they are still fairly high in calories and they should be consumed in moderation.

Whole Grains

Some whole grains are loaded with fiber and contain a decent amount of protein such as quinoa, oats, and brown rice. Oats, for example, contain beta-glucans – soluble fibers that have been shown to increase satiety and can boost metabolism.

Fruits

We all know that fruits are healthy. Studies have shown that people who eat the most fruits are healthier than those who don't. Although they contain natural sugar, fruits have a low energy density and take a while to chew. In addition to that, the fiber content helps prevent sugar from being released too quickly into our bloodstream.

Sardines

Sardines are oily fish that belongs to the most nutritious food you can eat. They contain sizeable amounts of nutrients that your body needs.

Shellfish

Shellfish contains equal nutrients as to organ meats. Some of the edible shellfish are clams, mollusks and oysters.

Shrimp

Shrimps are low in fat and calories but with high protein. They are also loaded with other nutrients such as selenium and Vitamin B12.

Brown rice

Rice is the staple food for more than half of the earth's population. It is the most popular cereal grains. Brown rice is equally nutritious which contains fiber, vitamin B1 and magnesium.

Oats

Oats are amazingly healthy. They are rich with nutrients and powerful fibers called beta glucans, which provide several benefits.

Quinoa

Quinoa is famous among individuals who are health-conscious. It is a tasty grain that is rich in nutrients such magnesium and fiber. Quinoa is also a major source of plant-based protein.

Coconut Oil

Coconut oil is high in fatty acids (medium-chain triglycerides) and these fatty acids help in boosting your satiety better than other fats.

Full-Fat Yogurt

There are certain types of yogurt that contain probiotic bacteria that can improve the function of our gut. A healthy gut helps protect against inflammation and leptin resistance that drives you away from being obese. But keep in mind that low-fat yogurt is loaded with sugar, so it's best if you avoid consuming it.

Cheese

Cheese is extremely nutritious. A single slice of cheese may offer the same amount of nutrients as a cup of milk. Aside from the fact that cheese is a delicious food that you can eat.

Whole milk

Milk is very high in mineral, vitamins, healthy fats and quality animal protein. It's also one of the best sources of calcium.

Butter (from grass-fed cows)

Butter which is from a grass-fed cow is high in many important nutrients like vitamin K2.

Potatoes

Potatoes are rich in potassium and contain a bit of every nutrient you need such as vitamin C. Potatoes can also keep you feel longer.

Sweet potatoes

Sweet potatoes are one the most delicious starchy foods that you can have. They're loaded with antioxidants and healthy nutrients.

Dark chocolate

Who says you cannot have chocolates? Almost everyone loves this sweet sinful thing. Dark chocolate is rich in magnesium and is known at the most powerful source of antioxidants.

There are lots of options in finding foods to stay healthy. Mainly, these foods are vegetables, fruit, nuts, seeds, legumes, like fish and lean meat. Certain processed foods, like probiotic yogurt, extra-virgin olive oil, and oatmeal are some of the best choices you can include. Furthermore, with regular exercise and moderation, eating these healthy and nutritious foods should help you to achieve a healthier life.

List of Unhealthy Foods to Avoid

After getting prepped up with all the health that we can have to stay fit and healthy, we seem to have overlooked the foods that are bad for us. The reason why it's hard for us to resist unhealthy food is that the things that make them bad is because they taste so good. Sweet, salty and fatty foods certainly taste good which a lot of us enjoy.

But we don't have to resort to living like a caveman. There are numerous types of foods that you can turn to taste good and won't risk your well-being. Here are some of the foods that we have to watch out for:

Fast Food

Fast food is bad for us, that is a given fact. The reason for this is because they use trans fats and additives to make the meals taste amazing. There are also tons of refined sugar, preservatives, and food coloring to make the food last longer.

Frozen Meals

We often choose to buy a quick and easy meal, especially when are too tired to prepare a meal. However, any of these frozen meals that are microwavable are loaded with hydrogenated oils, which contain trans-fat in some amount.

Trans-Fat Food

These is the most famous unhealthy ingredients that are present in our meals. Trans-fats are chemically made by the hydrogenation process which is hard for the body to digest. Research shows that trans-fat is connected to diabetes and obesity.

High Fructose Corn Syrup (HFCS)

Corn syrup has a strong appeal to us because it's not expensive, very sweet, and easy to store. Research shows that corn syrup causes metabolic dysregulation that leads to obesity.

Sweetened, Non-Organic Yogurt Foods

Although a lot of health-conscious add yogurt to their list of go-to food, the sweeteners it contains are to watch out for. Greek yogurt is the best kind of yogurt to have without all the added flavors or sugar.

Ketchup

Ketchup uses corn syrup. Stay away from French fries to avoid ketchup too!

Breakfast Cereals

Cereals have been the staple breakfast for most of us, especially for the kids. However, the popular brands of cereals contain high fructose corn syrup. Instead of cereals, try a bowl of oatmeal with fruits on top.

MSG (Monosodium Glutamate)

MSG is known to promote obesity, headaches, allergic reactions, liver inflammation, and even heart palpitations.

Ranch Dressing

You wouldn't have a salad without your dressing, right? But did you ever wonder why you can't get enough of this dressing? This salad dressing is loaded with artificial flavors and sweeteners that's why it tastes better.

Fried Foods

Most of us are already aware that fried foods are dangerous to our health. Fried foods contain high amounts of saturated fat, calories, trans fat, and cholesterol. Other than the fact that fried foods contain a high amount of MSG.

Packaged Salty Chips

The better tasting and more flavorings these packaged chips have, the more MSG and other artificial flavorings they contain. You can opt to make your own homemade chips using sweet potatoes and kales.

Artificial Sweeteners

These artificial sweeteners are like drugs that are addicting. However, the side effects include some really severe health conditions such as insomnia, blindness, hives, tinnitus, and depression. These conditions can also contribute to Alzheimer's.

Diet Colas and Sodas

Diet sodas sweeteners like aspartame. Research shows that aspartame is associated with a higher risk of dementia and stroke.

Packaged Diet Snacks

Many of these packaged snack packs are appealing to many dieters. But you should always opt to have whole foods versus packaged or processed foods.

Sodium Foods

Numerous amounts of sodium or salt are really dangerous to our health. Sodium foods cause us to retain water and it also increases blood pressure that can lead to complications with the heart.

Processed Cheese

Your favorite processed cheese contains a huge amount of sodium which is basically dangerous to your health.

Pizza

A slice of pizza contains a whole day's worth of sodium. And if you are getting toppings like sausage, ham, pepperoni, and other processed meats, you are doubling your sodium intake.

Cholesterol

There is good and bad cholesterol. Make sure to cut out from all the foods that contain any bad cholesterol.

Ice Cream

The famous comfort food whenever we experience emotional turmoil turns out as one of the foods that contain a high level of bad cholesterol.

Doughnuts

Doughnuts contain a combination of sugar, cholesterol, fat, and MSG with trans-fat. The cholesterol level of this sweet treat is pretty high.

Saturated Fat

Numerous studies have concluded that saturated fat is bad for us. Skip the animal fats and choose the healthier options like monounsaturated and polyunsaturated fatty acids.

Fast-food Burgers

Unfortunately, your ultimate favorite fast-food snack can wreak havoc on your health. These burgers contain high levels of saturated fat.

Calories

Foods that contain high in calories can really add an extra line to your waistline. If you don't watch your calorie intake, you won't even aware that you are consuming a lot.

Chocolate

Milk chocolate rules the market when it comes to a sweet treat. Maybe you are not aware of the high levels of sugar and calories contains on your favorite chocolate brand.

Carbohydrates

Foods that are high in carbohydrates are being digested quickly and tend to increase blood sugar levels. This will cause a release of insulin which will produce glycogen and get stored in our body as fat.

The Bottom Line

Health is most important for a good happy life. One cannot enjoy life without good health. Most important is taking care of your physical and emotional well-being.

Prevention is better than cure. Making healthy choices in life helps one remain healthy and have a better quality of life. People who don't take care of their health, and abuse their body by smoking, using drugs, drinking alcohol or overeating, end up with serious medical problems.

Health care costs are through the roof as people are not proactive in taking care of their health, and people wants the most advanced treatments when they suffer consequences of their poor unhealthy life choices.